49 Great Tasting Skin Cancer Juice Recipes:

Allow Your Skin to Fully Recover and Eliminate Cancer Cells Quickly and Naturally

By

Joe Correa CSN

COPYRIGHT

This publication is designed to provide accurate and authoritative information in regard to the subject matter covered. It is sold with the understanding that neither the author nor the publisher is engaged in rendering medical advice. If medical advice or assistance is needed, consult with a doctor. This book is considered a guide and should not be used in any way detrimental to your health. Consult with a physician before starting this nutritional plan to make sure it's right for you.

ACKNOWLEDGEMENTS

This book is dedicated to my friends and family that have had mild or serious illnesses so that you may find a solution and make the necessary changes in your life.

49 Great Tasting Skin Cancer Juice Recipes:

Allow Your Skin to Fully Recover and Eliminate Cancer Cells Quickly and Naturally

By

Joe Correa CSN

CONTENTS

ABOUT THE AUTHOR

After years of Research, I honestly believe in the positive effects that proper nutrition can have over the body and mind. My knowledge and experience has helped me live healthier throughout the years and which I have shared with family and friends. The more you know about eating and drinking healthier, the sooner you will want to change your life and eating habits.

Nutrition is a key part in the process of being healthy and living longer so get started today. The first step is the most important and the most significant.

INTRODUCTION

49 Great Tasting Skin Cancer Juice Recipes: Allow Your Skin to Fully Recover and Eliminate Cancer Cells Quickly and Naturally

By Joe Correa CSN

This book includes the best skin cancer preventive juices available to ensure your skin is strong and healthy in the least amount of time. Juicing is fast way to absorb essential cancer-fighting vitamins and minerals your body needs to protect itself from harmful toxins.

When it comes to preventing skin cancer, you might focus only on using sunscreen, a hat, long-sleeve shirts, or staying in the shade but you can still do much more. A diet rich in cancer-fighting vitamins and minerals can make a world of a difference when trying to prevent skin cancer.

To prevent and treat skin cancer it's crucial to maintain a healthy lifestyle (no alcohol, no smoking, doing exercise regularly and if possible outdoors, etc.) and a well-balanced diet. When trying to prevent or treat skin cancer, good eating habits can significantly reduce your chances of getting cancer or may at least help slow melanoma progression.

Foods rich in antioxidants, vitamins A, B, C, and D, and other compounds such as carotenoids, (especially beta-carotene) have proven to have many anti-carcinogenic properties that help to keep skin healthy and beautiful.

49 GREAT TASTING SKIN CANCER JUICE RECIPES: ALLOW YOUR SKIN TO FULLY RECOVER AND ELIMINATE CANCER CELLS QUICKLY AND NATURALLY

1.   PROTECTOR JUICE

In this juice, you will enjoy the perks of carotenoids such as alpha and beta-carotene found in carrots and the interactions of its components that make carrots a highly recommended vegetable for the prevention of many types of cancers such as skin cancer.

Ingredients:

- 2 Carrots, peeled
- 1 Apple
- 1 Celery stalk
- 1 tsp honey
- 1 cup water

Instructions:

- ✓ Wash the carrots, apple and celery stalk.
- ✓ Place all ingredients in a blender.

✓ Blend together while adding water until the desired consistency is reached.

2.   C+ POWER

Citric fruits are high in Vitamin C and other compounds that give them antioxidant properties. Also Vitamin C can reduce the negative sunburn reaction to UVB radiation, thus increasing the natural protective capabilities of our skin.

Ingredients:

- 1 cup Water
- 1 cup Green tea
- 1 Tamarillo
- ½ tsp Turmeric

Instructions:

- ✓ Wash tamarillo.
- ✓ Place all ingredients in a blender.
- ✓ Blend together while adding water until the desired consistency is reached.

3.   HYDRAJUICE

Green tea has many perks as it is well known for its antioxidant properties. Green tea contains catechins and other polyphenols, which have been related with anti-cancer properties and being able to protect your system from carcinogenic mutations.

Ingredients:

- 2 cups Green tea
- 1 cup diced watermelon
- 1 cup diced cantaloupe
- ¼ tsp ginger

Instructions:

- ✓ Place all ingredients in a blender.
- ✓ Blend together while adding water until the desired consistency is reached.

4.   BERRYLICIOUS

Blueberries and Raspberries are on the top of the list among antioxidants and anti-carcinogenic fruits; they have shown to contain a large variety of potent antitumor effects against cancer.

Ingredients:

- 2 cups Raspberries
- 1 cup Blueberries
- 2 Bananas
- 1 tsp cacao powder
- 2 cups coconut water

Instructions:

- ✓ Place all ingredients in a blender.
- ✓ Blend together while adding water until the desired consistency is reached.

5.   TROPIJUICY

Avocados are a great source of healthy omega-3 fatty acids, which are known to have anti-inflammatory properties and have been related to protective effects against cancer. Research also suggests that omega 3 fatty acids can help protect the skin from UV damage.

Ingredients:

- 1 Avocado, pitted and peeled
- 1 cup cherries, pitted
- 1 tsp cacao powder
- 1 tbsp coconut flakes
- 1 cup coconut water

Instructions:

- ✓ Place all ingredients in a blender.
- ✓ Blend together while adding water until the desired consistency is reached.

6.   VITALITY JUICE

Watercress is a good source of various vitamins like A, B and C vitamins. It has also been shown that Watercress reduces cancer risk, increases immune function, reduces blood cell DNA damage and has great antioxidant properties that will protect your skin from carcinogenic effects.

Ingredients:

- 2 cups Watercress
- ½ Cucumber
- 1 cup Strawberries
- 1 cup water

Instructions:

- ✓ Wash watercress and cucumber.
- ✓ Place all ingredients in a blender.
- ✓ Blend together while adding water until the desired consistency is reached.

7.   BERRY POWER

Grapes are highly recommended as they're a good source of resveratrol, which is a powerful antioxidant and is thought to help stop the aging process in humans, making them an excellent source for anti-cancer effects.

Ingredients:

- 1 cup Grapes
- 1 cup Raspberries
- ½ cup Pomegranate juice
- 1 cup diced Watermelon
- 1 cup water

Instructions:

- ✓ Wash grapes and raspberries.
- ✓ Place all ingredients in a blender.
- ✓ Blend together while adding water until the desired consistency is reached.

8.   SUPERKALE

Among the cruciferous vegetables, kale has the highest levels of vitamins. It is also a good source of carotenoids and phytonutrients which have been reported to have anti-cancer properties.

Ingredients:

- 2 cups Kale
- 1 cup diced Pineapple
- ¼ cup of Basil
- ½ cup lemon juice
- 1 cup water

Instructions:

- ✓ Wash kale leaves.
- ✓ Place all ingredients in a blender.
- ✓ Blend together while adding water until the desired consistency is reached.

9.   WILD-O-RADISH BOOSTER

The family of brassica vegetables is vast and horseradish is one of its members, as well as broccoli and kale. This family of vegetables is well-known for having components with cancer preventive properties.

Ingredients:

- 2 radish, sliced
- ½ cup broccoli head, chopped
- ½ cup kale
- 1 cup Pomegranate juice
- ¼ cup almonds

Instructions:

- ✓ Wash radish, broccoli and kale.
- ✓ Place all ingredients in a blender.
- ✓ Blend together while adding water until the desired consistency is reached.

10.   SUPER BERRYOCCOLI JUICE

Broccoli is highly recommended for a wide range of cancer and cardiovascular diseases. It's a good source of vitamins and substances that have been demonstrated for cancer-fighting properties and antioxidant protection.

Ingredients:

- 2 cup Broccoli heads, chopped
- 1 cup Blueberries
- 2 cups Grapefruit juice

Instructions:

- ✓ Wash blueberries and broccoli
- ✓ Place all ingredients in a blender.
- ✓ Blend together while adding water until the desired consistency is reached.

11.   MEGA-D

For this juice we want to enhance the properties of cherries by using Greek Yogurt, a natural source of vitamin D. There has been a lot of research on the relation between skin cancer and vitamin D., indicating that lower levels of vitamin D can be related to an increased risk of developing melanoma so let's boost up with the MEGA-D juice.

Ingredients:

- 2 cups Cherries
- 1 large Banana, peeled
- 2 dates
- 1 cup Greek Yoghurt

Instructions:

- ✓ Wash cherries.
- ✓ Place all ingredients in a blender.
- ✓ Blend together while adding water until the desired consistency is reached.

12.   SPICY JUICY

Spinach contains various carotenoids and lignans which have anti-carcinogenic properties. Add the cucurbitacins found in cucumbers that also provide anticancer effects, and this makes this juice highly recommended to keep your body hydrated and also prevent melanoma.

Ingredients:

- 2 cups Baby spinach leaves
- 1 cucumber, sliced
- ½ cup lemon juice
- 1 cup water
- ¼ tsp hot pepper

Instructions:

- ✓ Wash the cucumber and spinach.
- ✓ Place all ingredients in a blender.
- ✓ Blend together while adding water until the desired consistency is reached.

13. LYCOPENE BOOSTER

Tomatoes are full of goodness; they have shown to have antioxidant, anti-inflammatory, and cardio-protective properties. Several studies have found that greater consumption of tomatoes is associated with increased protection against sunburn and healthier skin.

Ingredients:

- 2 Tomatoes
- 1 Celery stalk
- 2 cups cranberry juice
- ¼ tsp Turmeric

Instructions:

- ✓ Wash the tomatoes and celery stalk.
- ✓ Place all ingredients in a blender.
- ✓ Blend together while adding water until the desired consistency is reached.

14. MELON MIX

The consumption of these melons -watermelon, cantaloupe, honeydew, - boost your system due to the high amount of carotenoids, which can help protect your skin against harmful ultraviolet radiation from the sun.

Ingredients:

- 1 cup diced Cantaloupe
- 1 cup diced Watermelon
- 1 cup diced Honeydew
- 1 cup water
- 1 tsp of lemon juice

Instructions:

- ✓ Place all ingredients in a blender.
- ✓ Blend together while adding water until the desired consistency is reached.

15. PINK JUICE

Guavas are a great source of beta-carotene and Vitamin C. Research has proven their chemopreventive effects, and also they are delicious, being one of the best fruits to start adding to your skin cancer preventive diet.

Ingredients:

- 2 Guavas, peeled
- 1 large Banana, peeled
- ½ cup cherries, pitted
- ½ cup strawberries
- 1 cup water

Instructions:

- ✓ Wash cherries and strawberries.
- ✓ Place all ingredients in a blender.
- ✓ Blend together while adding water until the desired consistency is reached.

16.   APRICOT SUNRISE

In this juice you can enjoy the benefits of carotenoids as well as vitamin D and selenium, a compound related to reducing the risk of developing melanoma.

Ingredients:

- 2 cups Apricot slices
- 1 large banana, peeled
- ½ cup rolled oats
- 1 cup almond milk
- 3 tbsp Greek yogurt

Instructions:

- ✓ Place all ingredients in a blender.
- ✓ Blend together while adding water until the desired consistency is reached.

17.   PURPLE BOOSTER

Pomegranates are an excellent source of chemopreventive compounds thanks to their polyphenols and lignans as these compounds are capable of inhibiting carcinogenic cells.

Ingredients:

- 1 cup Pomegranate juice
- 2 cups Grapes, seedless
- 1 cup Blueberries

Instructions:

- ✓ Wash grapes and berries.
- ✓ Place all ingredients in a blender.
- ✓ Blend together while adding water until the desired consistency is reached.

18.   SELENIUMIGHTY

Brazil nuts are among the greatest sources for Selenium. This mineral helps you protect your skin from sunburns, due to its properties to create antioxidant enzymes. Selenium also boosts the effectiveness of Vitamin C found in Kiwifruit.

Ingredients:

- ½ cup Brazil nuts
- 1 Banana, peeled
- 1 Kiwifruit, washed and sliced
- 1 Fig
- 1 cup water

Instructions:

- ✓ Place all ingredients in a blender.
- ✓ Blend together while adding water until the desired consistency is reached.

19.　BETA-DRINK

Mustard greens are a natural source of important nutrients as it contains beta-carotene, vitamin A, vitamin C, calcium and iron. It especially has high contents of beta-carotene, the well-known skin protector.

Ingredients:

- 1 cup Mustard greens
- 1 cup chopped Mango
- ½ cup cherries
- 1 tsp lemon juice
- 1 cup water

Instructions:

- ✓ Wash mustard greens and cherries.
- ✓ Place all ingredients in a blender.
- ✓ Blend together while adding water until the desired consistency is reached.

20.   GREEN ENERGY

Romaine lettuce is one of the most nutritious among all the lettuces. It contains great amounts of beta-carotene, lutein and vitamin K.

Ingredients:

- 2 cups Romaine Lettuce
- 1 Cucumber, sliced
- 1 cup chopped Pineapple
- 1 tsp lemon juice
- 1 cup water

Instructions:

- ✓ Wash romaine lettuce and cucumber.
- ✓ Place all ingredients in a blender.
- ✓ Blend together while adding water until the desired consistency is reached.

21. SUNSET JUICE

The compounds that give the orange-yellowish common coloration of apricots, peaches and pumpkins also provide anti-carcinogenic properties. Combine this with the many properties of turmeric, such as antioxidant, anti-inflammatory, and antibacterial effects, and you have a wonderful juice to prevent cancer.

Ingredients:

- 1 cup pumpkin purée
- 1 cup chopped peach
- 1 cup chopped apricot
- ½ tsp turmeric
- 1 cup water
- 4 walnuts, chopped

Instructions:

- ✓ Place all ingredients in a blender.
- ✓ Blend together while adding water until the desired consistency is reached.

22. BROBOOST

In this smoothie we are combining so much power. We will find Bromelain properties from the pineapples, plus carotenoids and antioxidants from spinach. All of these compounds give your body a great source of anti-cancer nutrients.

Ingredients:

- 1 cup chopped Pineapple fruit
- 2 cups Baby Spinach leaves
- ½ tsp ginger
- 1 cup water

Instructions:

- ✓ Wash the baby spinach leaves.
- ✓ Place all ingredients in a blender.
- ✓ Blend together while adding water until the desired consistency is reached.

23. K+AID

Flaxseeds have a substantial amount of healthy omega-3 fatty acids. As cancer-preventive compounds, these healthy omega-3 fatty acids play an important role in regulating our immune system, which is a valuable role when aiming to prevent carcinogenic cells appearing in our bodies.

Ingredients:

- ½ cup flaxseeds
- 1 cup chopped apricots
- 1 Green apple, sliced
- 1 cup water

Instructions:

- ✓ Wash the green apple.
- ✓ Place all ingredients in a blender.
- ✓ Blend together while adding water until the desired consistency is reached.

24. JUICYMINT

Let's highlight the benefits of raspberries: they are an incredible source of diverse phytochemicals, including ellagic acid and anthocyanin, both of which have shown to inhibit cancer cell growth.

Ingredients:

- 1 cup Raspberries
- 1 banana, peeled
- ¼ tsp Mint leaves
- 1 cup water

Instructions:

- ✓ Wash the raspberries.
- ✓ Place all ingredients in a blender.
- ✓ Blend together while adding water until the desired consistency is reached.

25. ORIENTAL JUICE

Watermelon is also highly recommended for skin cancer prevention, because is an excellent source of carotenoids, L-citrulline, and cucurbitacins. These compounds have been shown to have chemopreventive properties so we have a delicious and nutritious juice.

Ingredients:

- 1 cup cubed watermelon
- 1 Kiwi, peeled, cubed
- 1 cup Green Tea
- 1 tsp honey

Instructions:

- ✓ Wash kiwi then peel and cube.
- ✓ Place all ingredients in a blender.
- ✓ Blend together while adding water until the desired consistency is reached.

26. JUPITER BERRIES

Berries rank among the highest of all fruits and vegetables in their properties against cancer. Blueberries have amazing properties, including the ability to destroy free radicals, and to show neuroprotective and cardioprotective properties.

Ingredients:

- 1 cup Strawberries
- 1 cup Blueberries
- 1 cup Cherries
- 1 cup water

Instructions:

- ✓ Wash all the berries.
- ✓ Place all ingredients in a blender.
- ✓ Blend together while adding water until the desired consistency is reached.

27. YELLOWISH

Turmeric has so many benefits as an antioxidant, anti-inflammatory, antibacterial, neuroprotective and cardio-protective compound. Some research has also shown that turmeric has a variety of anti-cancer properties against a wide range of cancers.

Ingredients:

- ½ tsp turmeric
- 1 cup chopped Papaya
- 1 cup chopped Mango
- 1 tsp lemon juice
- 1 cup water

Instructions:

- ✓ Place all ingredients in a blender.
- ✓ Blend together while adding water until the desired consistency is reached.

28.   LIFE-ENHANCING

Mangos are full of vitamins and beta-carotene, while blueberries and raspberries are well-known for its phytochemicals compounds that give them excellent anti-cancer properties.

Ingredients:

- 1 cup Mango slices
- 1 cup cherries, pitted
- 1 Fig
- 1 cup Broccoli florets
- 1 cup water

Instructions:

- ✓ Wash the cherries and broccoli florets.
- ✓ Place all ingredients in a blender.
- ✓ Blend together while adding water until the desired consistency is reached.

29. HOLY JUICE

Pineapples have a unique compound which is been reported to have many anti-cancer properties called bromelain. This compound has pro-apoptic, anti-invasive and anti-metastatic properties so very useful in preventing skin cancer.

Ingredients:

- 2 cups chopped pineapple
- 1 green apple
- ½ sliced cucumber
- ½ tsp Ginger
- 1 cup water

Instructions:

- ✓ Wash the cucumber and apple.
- ✓ Place all ingredients in a blender.
- ✓ Blend together while adding water until the desired consistency is reached.

30.   GRAN-AID

Research shows the anti-carcinogenic properties of pomegranate, as it is shown to inhibit the growth of skin cancer tumors. It also has chemopreventive properties so drinking pomegranate juice often can help stay away from skin cancer.

Ingredients:

- 2 cups chopped Honeydew
- 1 Kiwi, sliced
- 1 cup Pomegranate juice

Instructions:

- ✓ Wash kiwi then slice.
- ✓ Place all ingredients in a blender.
- ✓ Blend together while adding water until the desired consistency is reached.

31. SWISSBOOST

Swiss chard is one of the healthiest vegetables available. It is a terrific source of antioxidants and anti-inflammatory compounds such as beta-carotene, lutein, zeaxanthin, Kaempferol, and quercetin, which can play a promoting role in your body's defenses and skin health.

Ingredients:

- 1 cup Swiss chard
- 1 cup chopped Pineapple
- ½ cup cherries, pitted
- ½ cup blueberries
- 1 cup water

Instructions:

- ✓ Wash cherries and blueberries.
- ✓ Place all ingredients in a blender.
- ✓ Blend together while adding water until the desired consistency is reached.

32.   VITATURNIP

Thanks to the large amount of Vitamin A found in turnip greens, they are really good for your skin and hair health. They also have high amounts of vitamin C to help with building and repairing of collagen tissue in our skin.

Ingredients:

- 1 cup Turnip greens
- 1 Cucumber, sliced
- 1 cup Pomegranate juice
- ½ tsp ginger

Instructions:

- ✓ Wash turnip greens and cucumber.
- ✓ Place all ingredients in a blender.
- ✓ Blend together while adding water until the desired consistency is reached.

33.   NATURAL POWER

Almonds can help maintain your skin health. They're a great source of Vitamin E and other antioxidants that help in nourishing your skin. In some research, there are even indications that eating almonds can help our bodies fight skin cancer and reverse oxidative damages.

Ingredients:

- 8 almonds
- 1 cup blueberries
- 1 cup Strawberries
- 1 cup Greek Yoghurt
- ¼ tsp fresh Mint

Instructions:

- ✓ Wash the blueberries and strawberries.
- ✓ Place all ingredients in a blender.
- ✓ Blend together while adding water until the desired consistency is reached.

34.   D-TOX

Pistachios are a fabulous nut to include in our juices and meals. They contain a high amount of lutein and zeaxanthin, which have shown to improve your health and decrease the risk of cancer, particularly skin and eye diseases.

Ingredients:

- ½ cup pistachios, shelled
- 1 Carrot
- 1 Cucumber
- 1 cup Grapes
- 1 cup water

Instructions:

- ✓ Wash the carrot, cucumber and grapes.
- ✓ Place all ingredients in a blender.
- ✓ Blend together while adding water until the desired consistency is reached.

35. OLYMJUS

Cacao powder is the original source of most chocolates we eat every day. Cacao powder is the best way to get all of the benefits from chocolate, as it contains a higher quantity of phytonutrients. Chocolate even has more antioxidants than tea, so it's better at reducing the risk of developing cancer.

Ingredients:

- 2 tbsp Cacao powder
- ½ Avocado, pitted, peeled
- 1 cup raspberries
- 1 cup Water
- 5 Almonds

Instructions:

- ✓ Place all ingredients in a blender.
- ✓ Blend together while adding water until the desired consistency is reached.

36.   CAROTEN-AID

Sunflower seeds are a perfect snack for your health. They help prevent cancer due to their high antioxidant content and they are a great source of selenium, a compound which has been found to have anti-cancer effects such as stimulating cancer cell apoptosis.

Ingredients:

- 2 tbsp Sunflower seeds
- ½ cup Pumpkin puree
- 1 cup apricot, sliced
- ½ tsp turmeric
- 1 cup water

Instructions:

- ✓ Place all ingredients in a blender.
- ✓ Blend together while adding water until the desired consistency is reached.

37.   VITAGOJILIN

Goji berries supply us with high levels of antioxidants, vitamin C, and vitamin A. All these nutrients are key in helping our immune system stay strong and prevent illnesses, ranging from a common cold to a chronic, dangerous disease like cancer. Goji berries promote healthy skin and act like a natural preventive measure against skin cancer.

Ingredients:

- 1 cup Goji Berries
- 1 cup Grapes
- 1 cup Coconut water
- 1 tbsp Flaxseed

Instructions:

- ✓ Wash grapes and goji berries.
- ✓ Place all ingredients in a blender.
- ✓ Blend together while adding water until the desired consistency is reached.

38.   GRAPE GOODIE

Grapes are full of nutrients and vitamins, and phytonutrients like resveratrol that has been linked to anti-cancer effects on a variety of cancers. Grapes also provide us with beta-carotene, flavonoids, and antioxidants, which means that grapes are an incredible cancer-fighting food.

Ingredients:

- 1 cup grapes, seedless
- 1 banana
- 1 cup Cherries, pitted
- 1 cup Pomegranate juice

Instructions:

- ✓ Wash grapes and cherries.
- ✓ Place all ingredients in a blender.
- ✓ Blend together while adding water until the desired consistency is reached.

39. GREENS'N'BERRIES

Blackberries are ranked among the highest antioxidant foods. This tells us that eating more Blackberries -and most berries in general- can help your system eliminate free radicals and prevent the proliferation of carcinogenic cells.

Ingredients:

- 1 cup Blackberries
- 1 cup Strawberries
- 1 cup Broccoli florets
- 1 tsp honey
- 1 cup water

Instructions:

- ✓ Wash the blackberries, strawberries and broccoli florets.
- ✓ Place all ingredients in a blender.
- ✓ Blend together while adding water until the desired consistency is reached.

40.   FIGFIGHTER

Figs and fig leaves are natural cancer-fighting foods. Figs contain powerful antioxidants, which have shown to be very effective to combat various types of cancer. More specifically, fig leaves can help prevent skin cancer due to its natural free radical damage fighters.

Ingredients:

- 2 Figs
- ¼ cup Fig leaves
- 1 cup chopped Papaya
- 1 cup chopped Mango, peeled and pitted
- 1 cup Greek yogurt

Instructions:

- ✓ Wash mango and fig leaves.
- ✓ Place all ingredients in a blender.
- ✓ Blend together while adding water until the desired consistency is reached.

41.   CITRUS INFUSION

Pomegranates are a good source of chemopreventive compounds, thanks to their polyphenols and lignans. These compounds are capable of inhibiting cancer cell proliferation and promote apoptosis.

Ingredients:

- 1 cup Pomegranate juice
- 2 grapefruits
- 1 cup diced Pineapple
- 1 tsp honey

Instructions:

- ✓ Wash the grapefruits and squeeze juice.
- ✓ Place all ingredients in a blender.
- ✓ Blend together while adding water until the desired consistency is reached.

42. GREENIE

Matcha is the end-product of ground and processed green tea, but this powder has about 10 times the amount of antioxidants compared to green tea. Many studies have demonstrated the incredible effectiveness of matcha to prevent cancers of all sorts.

Ingredients:

- 1 tsp Matcha
- 1 Avocado, pitted, peeled
- ½ cup cherries, pitted
- 1 Celery stalk
- 1 cup water

Instructions:

- ✓ Wash the cherries and celery stalk.
- ✓ Place all ingredients in a blender.
- ✓ Blend together while adding water until the desired consistency is reached.

43.   O'FIG'IN

In this juice we are obtaining the properties of blueberries, almonds, figs and watermelon. All of these ingredients are well-known for their anti-cancer effects due to their high levels of vitamins and nutrients. With this powerful juice you can nourish your body and protect your skin.

Ingredients

- 1 cup Blueberries
- 1 Fig
- 1 cup chopped watermelon
- 5 almonds
- 1 cup water

Instructions:

✓ Wash the blueberries.

✓ Place all ingredients in a blender.

✓ Blend together while adding water until the desired consistency is reached.

44. SUNNY CHERRY JUICE

Sunny cherry juice is not only a tasty and wonderful juice but also an incredible source of vitamins and nutrients with many chemopreventive properties. We can see from the main ingredient – cherries - we obtain the flavonoids that give them their intense red coloration and possess these compounds with antioxidant, anti-inflammatory and cancer-preventing properties.

Ingredients:

- 2 cups cherries
- 1 cup diced Mango
- 1 cup chopped pineapple
- 1 cup Pomegranate juice

Instructions:

- ✓ Wash the cherries, mango and pineapple.
- ✓ Place all ingredients in a blender.
- ✓ Blend together while adding water until the desired consistency is reached.

45.   RISE'N'SHINE

Levels in blood of Vitamin D can be highly related to chances to get skin cancer. An important source of Vitamin D for our bodies is actually the sun, but extended exposure to the sun can negatively affect your skin. For this reason, we bring you the Rise'n'Shine juice that provides vitamin D from another source such as fortified Almond Milk.

Ingredients:

- 1 cup vitamin D fortified Almond milk
- 1 Banana, peeled
- 2 tbsp Flaxseed
- 4 almonds

Instructions:

- ✓ Place all ingredients in a blender.
- ✓ Blend together while adding water until the desired consistency is reached.

46.   WAKE ME UP

Chia seeds have grown to be a very popular ingredient in health snacks as research has proven that chia seeds supply a very high amount of antioxidants so they can help speed up the skin's repair and prevent further damages, such as skin cancer.

Ingredients:

- 2 tbsp Chia seeds
- 1 banana, peeled
- 1 cup chopped Pineapple
- 1 tsp honey
- 1 cup water

Instructions:

- ✓ Place all ingredients in a blender.
- ✓ Blend together while adding water until the desired consistency is reached.

47. CHOCOPOW

This juice will bring a lot of vitamin and nutrients, including the omega-3 fatty acids from the walnuts, the phytonutrients from cherries, the antioxidants from Cacao powder and many Vitamins com the almond milk; all of these in a delicious juice.

Ingredients:

- 4 Walnuts
- 1 cup cherries, pitted
- 1 tbsp Cacao powder
- 1 cup Almond milk

Instructions:

- ✓ Wash the cherries.
- ✓ Place all ingredients in a blender.
- ✓ Blend together while adding water until the desired consistency is reached.

48.   OXIJUICE

Tamarillo, or tree tomato, is an exotic and incredibly healthy fruit with high levels of vitamins and nutrients. With your aim to protect your skin and prevent skin cancer, this juice has to become part of your usual drinks.

Ingredients:

- 2 tamarillo, peeled
- 1 cup Green tea
- 1 cup strawberries

Instructions:

- ✓ Wash the tamarillo and strawberries.
- ✓ Place all ingredients in a blender.
- ✓ Blend together while adding water until the desired consistency is reached.

49. MANGOODISH

Mangos are full of vitamins and beta-carotene. These compounds give mangos their anti-aging attributes, combined with their high levels of vitamins A and C, mangos even help to build collagen, repair skin damages, and prevent skin cancer.

Ingredients:

- 1 cup chopped mango
- 1 cup green tea
- ½ cup blueberries
- 1 tsp turmeric

Instructions:

✓ Wash the blueberries.

✓ Place all ingredients in a blender.

✓ Blend together while adding water until the desired consistency is reached.

ADDITIONAL TITLES FROM THIS AUTHOR

70 Effective Meal Recipes to Prevent and Solve Being Overweight: Burn Fat Fast by Using Proper Dieting and Smart Nutrition

By

Joe Correa CSN

48 Acne Solving Meal Recipes: The Fast and Natural Path to Fixing Your Acne Problems in Less Than 10 Days!

By

Joe Correa CSN

41 Alzheimer's Preventing Meal Recipes: Reduce or Eliminate Your Alzheimer's Condition in 30 Days or Less!

By

Joe Correa CSN

70 Effective Breast Cancer Meal Recipes: Prevent and Fight Breast Cancer with Smart Nutrition and Powerful Foods

By

Joe Correa CSN